Powerlifting for the People

Table of Contents

Introduction

For decades, sports have dominated the country. Now-a-days, every major television channel airs sporting games and events year-round. This includes professional sports, as well as sports on the high school level. Some networks air sporting events that are on the junior high age level. Outside of television, magazines and newspapers have also joined the sport's frenzy. Conversations pertaining to a particular sport can be heard on a daily basis in the workplace, at schools and colleges, hospitals, corporate events, beauty shops/spas, and a host of other places. The attention of viewers was originally consumed with baseball, basketball, and football, but as the years go by, viewers have begun to focus their attention on other sports, including powerlifting. This sport is quickly coming into the picture, and it is going to stick around for decades to come.

Powerlifting is a sport that has no real age-barrier; people between the ages of 13 and 70 have been seen powerlifting around the world. This sport is fun and physically challenging. Even though powerlifting is not a new sport, it will make a huge impact over the next few years. There has even been talk for many years of powerlifting potentially going into the Olympics. Powerlifting has been shown on television occasionally, as well some of the big meets being live streamed over the internet, across huge platforms; this sport is quickly making its way into the public's eye. Many schools around the world are beginning to accept powerlifting as a club sport, in both high schools and colleges across the country.

Powerlifting has many advantages, and *one of the best is that is doesn't discriminate people of different shapes and sizes*. So many people opt out of participating in a sport because they are not the right height or size; however, there is no height requirement to become a powerlifter. Another common misconception about powerlifting is that you need to be a huge person. There are weight classes for every size; even a 97-pound class for and up to 308 pounds and Super Heavies for the men. So no matter how big you are, powerlifting has a class for you. The sport is open to anyone that is willing to try. Powerlifting does require dedication, strength, and the ability to train hard. Training for powerlifting is just as intense as any other sport. It requires an emotional, mental, and physical strength. The fact is, an athlete will get out of powerlifting what he or she puts into it. When athletes put in more, the better their rewards will be. You will be able to adapt to the sport better. You also have the potential to compete, successfully.

With thousands of powerlifters competing on an international level – as well as thousands of professional competitors within the United States – this sport is definitely here to stay, and will increase popularity each year.

Chapter 1: Strength Training

Powerlifting is a strength sport, but strength goes beyond the sport itself. Most people are under the misconception that strength is determined by how strong a person is... This is not entirely true. You may picture a bodybuilder with huge biceps and muscles bulging out all over their body. Perhaps an athlete or a person with great weight lifting capabilities pops into your mind when you hear the word strength. The truth is that strength is just as much a mental aspect as it is a physical attribute. Strength also pertains to your mental and emotional being. When you have the ability to overcome obstacles, large and small, you have great strength. If there are tasks that seem insurmountable, but you take them on anyway, you are showing great strength.

In all aspects of your life, you will need to have strength, not just the physical tasks you take on every day. In order to be successful at whatever you are doing, strength is required. If you want to achieve a better you – a more explosive you – it is important to have strength. Being strong in many areas could help you achieve the things that you set out to accomplish. If you are playing a sport, you will need to have mental and physical strength. As an athlete, the more strength that you have, the better you will perform. The same type of strength is required when you want to be promoted at your job. If you are a strong performer, and have the strength to handle the tasks handed down to you, this could lead to a promotion or better job offer with another company.

The bottom line is that the more strength you have, the stronger you are. The stronger you are emotionally, physically, and mentally, the more likely you are to accomplish the things that you want to achieve in life. It is important that athletes and individuals who are training take that strength they are building inside of the gym, and apply it to their daily performances and obstacles outside of the gym. This helps your overall spiritual well-being.

It is important to look at strength through many eyes. When you are working or training, it is important that you know how much you can handle, and what you cannot. This applies to both lifting, and in life. If it isn't a competition or game day most of the time, you should leave a little in "the tank." This way, you have some left in your reserve for another day. If you constantly go for broke every single workout, or in your everyday life - be it your job or something else - when you need that reserve, you won't have it. Let's say you are part of a big company or you run a business… If you need to delegate projects to other group members, you should do so. This will allow you to be more productive, and get more out of your day. Your body tells you what you are strong enough to handle. This does not mean you have given in, or up; instead, you have chosen not to over-extended yourself. The same applies to weight lifting, sports, and general fitness. When your body tells you enough is enough, you need to be strong enough to stop. This does not signal defeat; it signals strength. You are strong enough to do what you can, and strong enough to build up to doing more. Doing too much could be bad for your physical and mental being. When you are truly physically and emotionally strong, you will find a balance. You will learn when it is time to push, and when it is time to take a break and shut it down. Mastering yourself, along with your mind and body, is one of the truest signs of strength.

There is nothing wrong with adding on another five pounds here and there during strength training, but there is something wrong with adding too many pounds that could potentially place you in the hospital. There is nothing strong about causing harm to yourself, so do not do it. Small progression, overtime, is the healthiest and smartest approach to help prevent this. Many people try to rush the process by trying to do too much, too soon. Remember the story of the Tortoise and the Hare? Slow and steady wins the race. If you are trying to skip steps and make gains too quickly, this can lead to injury and burn out. Taking your time and being patient is a much healthier and sound approach to lifting, and life. Know your limits, and know how far to push them without injuring yourself. This doesn't mean you should not push yourself; it means you should do so in a controlled, systematic way. Steady consistency over a long period of time will always win over a very high-paced effort in the short-run. Think of it like a marathon versus a sprint. If you try to go fast at the start of a marathon you will use up all of your energy and not be able to finish. You will need to pace yourself and conserve your energy along the way, in order to finish. There will be times when you will need to push harder when the race is going uphill, and other times when you have to coast and the course is going down hill. Again, a consistent pace over the entire race will yield the best time, just like consistent practice over time will yield the best result.

It is easier for a competitive lifter or performance athlete to measure strength, in comparison to someone who is not either of the two. However, strength training is there to help you measure your strengths correctly. As you get stronger mentally, you can accurately measure your physicality. When you are mentally prepared to add weight to the bar, you can physically do so.

The goal that you have set will help you increase your strength. If you want to get stronger, you will need to work hard, consistently over time, in order to see that happens physically. However, if you just want to feel better about yourself, mentally and emotionally, strength training will help you with that accomplishment. Regardless if your goal is to be a competitive lifter, you can train hard to get stronger in order to achieve that goal.

Strength training is extremely important, regardless if you are a competitive lifter or just doing it to get stronger. The training can help with your endurance, and overall performance. It also helps you prevent injuries; even though more athletes have been injured playing football and soccer than people who participate in powerlifting.

Whatever your goal is, strength training will help you prepare to achieve it. You can get faster, stronger, and wiser – helping you improve the qualities and goals that you have set in place.

Testimonial:

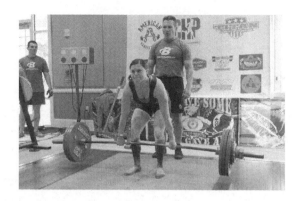

"Powerlifting has become so much more than a hobby. It is something I believe has played a crucial role in the person I have become. My training sessions challenge me physically and mentally. Fighting through tough workouts has helped shape me into a stronger person. As a woman, I am constantly hearing the negatives as for why women should not lift, especially not heavy. I, however, see no negatives in challenging the body and mind to become a better, stronger individual. The weights provide a judgment free outlet that either sex can benefit from. Plus, if you are lucky enough to find a team as amazing as the one I have found in Gaglione Strength, you will become a part of something much more.

It is an amazing feeling to be part a group of individuals that come together to help push one another to become better in and out of the gym." - *Ashlyn DiNinni*

Chapter 2: Benefits of Powerlifting

There are many reasons why people choose to lift, and the benefits associated with this sport are just some of those reasons. If you are looking to build muscle and improve your body composition, this is the sport for you. Powerlifting also has the potential to help you improve your athletic ability while burning off fat.

The sport of powerlifting is actually three lifts:

- Squat
- Bench Press
- DeadLift

In competition, these three lifts are used to determine your entire body strength. The squat is used to measure your lower body and your core strength. The bench press is used to measure your upper body strength and your pressing muscles. The deadlift is the lift that will measure your overall body strength and pulling muscles. When you do the deadlift, it will work with your legs, as well as your pulling muscles of the upper body as well as your core. When you combine all three of these lifts in a workout, you have the benefit of working out every muscle within your body. This is beneficial if you just want a good workout, if you have a weight loss goal, if you want to build muscle, or if you just want to experience peace of mind.

With an athlete, powerlifting helps you gain strength. You will become stronger all over, and you will achieve a bigger foundation for other athletic qualities. If you want to become more powerful, faster, or more explosive, powerlifting could help you achieve these facets. For example, if you are a runner, your absolute strength would require your legs to be measured in a squat. The stronger your squat is, the stronger your overall leg strength is going to be. This is great for a runner, because he or she will use a lower percentage of energy each time they take a stride. The stronger your body is, the more efficient you become. When you improve your overall strength, you could gain speed or more endurance; whatever it is that you have set out to achieve.

Powerlifting could also help an athlete improve his vertical jump. There is a <> correlation between the vertical leap and squat strength. If your goal is jump higher, you will need to build a bigger squat through powerlifting. You are building strength in your legs and hips, which both of which has the ability to help you improve your vertical jump, in addition to many other physical activities and sports. Combat sports in particular require a great deal of strength, particularly relative strength. Relative strength means that you need to be strong "pound for pound," in other words strong for your size. Some of those sports include wrestling, martial arts, and competitive fighting. Regardless if your athletic goal is endurance or power, having more strength will provide a larger foundation so there is more potential for growth and achievement in other athletic endeavors.

Athletes that participate in other sports will often lift to help prevent injuries. Powerlifting can help you reduce the amount of risks that are associated with physical activities, as well as sporting activities. It is true that the benefits associated with powerlifting go well beyond those associated with conventional lifting.

So many people want to improve their overall physique; therefore, they turn to powerlifting. If you are one of these people, lifting could help you with fat loss. Powerlifting is an intense form of exercise that helps you burn a lot of calories since the powerlifts are compound movements that utilize a lot of muscle groups simultaneously. The benefits do not stop with burning calories now; powerlifting can help with your long-term appearance as well. It has a long-term effect on your metabolism. Powerlifting is very effective when your goal is to drop fat and preserve lean muscle tissue when dieting since you are engaging a great deal of muscle mass when performing the three powerlifts.

There are benefits associated with powerlifting that have nothing to do with an athlete or competitor. Perhaps you are someone who just wants to get better, in regards to your appearance or physique. When you take up powerlifting, you have the benefit of building on your foundation to improve your muscles. The more strength you have, the more potential you have at using a higher volume, pertaining to squats, bench pressing, and dead lifts. This will allow for great potential growth for added muscle mass across your entire body

There are health issues and illnesses that powerlifting has the potential to help with, such as skeletal health. One out of every five women within the United States will be diagnosed with osteoporosis. Resistance training has the potential to combat the onset of osteoporosis by increasing bone mineral density. Powerlifting also increases strength and bone mass, which helps decrease the amount of risk factors that are associated with osteoporosis.

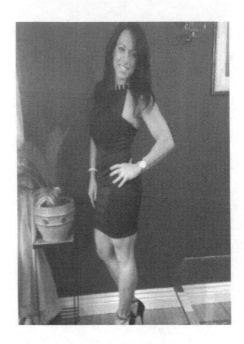

Testimonial:

"As a mother of 3 young boys, and currently being in remission from Grave's disease, it is imperative for me to keep my stress levels down. In my quest to reduce stress, I discovered a side of myself that I never knew I had . It is through Gaglione Strength that I found my true passion when it comes to strength training. At 39 years old, I competed in my first powerlifting event. I was never involved in sports growing up, and never competed in anything in my life, so for me this was a really big deal. I must admit I was reluctant at first, but it only took a couple of training sessions for me to realize that this is it!! This is where I need to be!!! I am honored to be part of such an amazing powerlifting team.

This sport has done more for me than most people realize, and for that, I will be forever grateful!" – *Laura*

Chapter 3: The Myths Behind Powerlifting

There are many misconceptions pertaining to powerlifting. In fact, lots of people shy away from powerlifting due to the myths behind the sport. With so many "experts" stating opinion, many people take those words as facts. In reality, they are myths.

The first myth is that powerlifting is only for people who are big and strong. The truth is that powerlifting is for anyone who wants to do it. While it is true that you have to be committed to the sport, it is something that anyone with a strong will can do. In fact, you can begin with an empty bar, or a simple broomstick. All you need to do is work on your squat, bench press, and deadlift. You do not need to be able to do a certain poundage to be considered a powerlifter, you just need to do the competition exercises and compete. Powerlifters come in all types of shapes, sizes, and strength levels.

Another myth is that children and elderly individuals cannot participate in powerlifting. While you may not see a five or six year old lifting weights, it is not uncommon for teens to powerlift. There are teen divisions pertaining to powerlifting, meaning that people begin training for the sport early on. As far as elderly individuals, some people over the age of 60 enjoy powerlifting. If your body is in good shape, you can participate in the sport at an older age. You do not want to overdo it, which is why you should always know your physical and mental strength.

Another myth associated with powerlifting is that muscle turns to fat when you stop lifting. If muscle turned to fat instantly, that would be a great magic trick. Being truthful, it just doesn't happen like that. Fat does not turn into muscle, and muscle does not turn into fat. Having more muscle mass can have a positive effect on your metabolism, which will allow you to burn fat. The more you work out and lift, the more calories you will burn off. Having increase muscle mass can help you burn off fat, and that muscle does not turn into flab if you decide to take a break from lifting. However, you will need to continue exercising on a regular basis to maintain good health, and your current state of fitness.

One of the most fraudulent myths associated with powerlifting is that the more you lift, the more results you see. Your workout should contain bodyweight exercises, in addition to heavy and light weights. Lifting lighter weights for high volume can be just as effective for your body as doing reps with heavy weights with lower volume. Of course, depending on your goal, and if you are getting ready for a competition certain types of workouts will help with certain goals. High volume and moderate weights are great for building strength, muscle mass, and building up work capacity, as well as conditioning. Lower volume and heavy weights are great for testing and peaking your strength for a competition. Lifting weights fast, with a light weight for low reps, is great for building up speed and explosive power. This is why it is important to utilize workouts that incorporate all types of workouts so you get the benefit from each method. The key factor in this scenario is that you lift until you have reached your goal for the day – or until you are fatigue. The point is that heavy weights all the time is not always the answer. There are times to lift heavy and there are times to lift lighter loads. Both have their place and can help build strength.

Some people are under the misconception that weight lifting causes high blood pressure. This is a myth. Yes, your blood pressure will be raised quite a bit during your actual lifting (especially during max weights), which is probably where the myth comes from, but this will not inherently raise your blood pressure during everyday life. In the past, people who were diagnosed with hypertension were told not to lift weights, but the truth is that powerlifting and aerobics can lower blood pressure. Both dialostic and systolic can be lowered due to powerlifting. The American Heart Association states that a person only has to put in two or three sessions a week, in order to begin seeing positive results.

Do not rely heavily on machines when exercising. So many people believe that machines are more effective than free weights. The truth is when you lift free weights, this activity mimics natural movement and it creates greater muscle activity, in comparison to machines. When you lift free weights, more muscles are recruited, which leads to greater strength gains. The reason is that free weights require you to stabilize the weight and machines stabilize the weight for you. The other benefit to free weights versus machines is that you are not locked into a specific position and you can move the way your body wants to. A machine locks you in a position that might be good or bad for your body, but when using free weights you can find the position that works best for your body. Weighted squats produce more muscle activity when compared to squats using a machine.

One of the biggest myths associated with powerlifting is that it makes you more susceptible to injuries>. The truth is, powerlifting does not make you prone to injury. This too is a misconception that many people have. When you have a good coach who can teach you the proper mechanics, you will know how to lift with the proper form. For example, as long as you are lifting with a braced neutral spine, keeping your back in a good position, keeping your knees in a good alignment, keeping your wrists and elbows in good alignment, getting stronger is actually very, very beneficial for preventing injuries, helping prevent muscle strains, and other things similar to that.

Do not shy away from powerlifting because you think it is a costly activity. The truth is that powerlifting is very affordable. If you are just starting out, you can actually visit a commercial gym that has barbell and plates to begin. There are not many monetary roadblocks when it pertains to powerlifting. This sport is something that is accessible to everyone. There are many platforms available for people wanting to train. There are also affordable coaches available to you as well.

Testimonial:

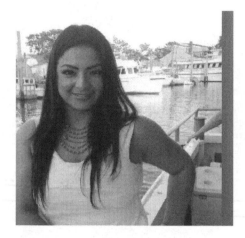

"Powerlifting has been one of the most beautiful experiences in my life! I've always been into sports; before I did gymnastics, Zumba, kickboxing and also running. I didn't really know much about powerlifting .I used to see those big guys on TV competing and I used think, it's super cool! I never thought it was possible to actually do it. The concept of powerlifting is amazing. The personal challenge of strength, focused and progression, is what makes powerlifting the most interesting and addictive sport in the world to me. I used to come and see my boyfriend, Mark, train, and sometimes I wondered if one day in the future I would be able to lift heavy weights like him. Lol!

One big day, thank God, I had the opportunity to go to see my boyfriend Mark competing with some of the strongest people in powerlifting – it took place at Raw Unity 7. It was a completely life-changing for me; I was able to see other competitors, both men and women!! I was ecstatic to be surrounded by such strong athletes, and ever since that weekend, my life changed, all because I wanted to lift and lift, lol! More important to me are the people I have around me. I feel blessed to have found the most professional coaches and instructors. In fact, this could never, ever, ever be possible without a good coach like John Gaglione. I've been learning each more and more each day. I feel mentally and physically stronger than ever, and this is a great feeling… the feeling of power lifting.

Thank you so much John for teaching me to be the best in life!" – *Bianca Vega*

Chapter 4: Powerlifting and the Athlete

Everyone takes up the sport of powerlifting for different reasons; therefore, the effect that powerlifting has on individuals will vary. If you are an athlete who powerlifts, your goals are different from those who simply want to have a better physique. The benefits of powerlifting will vary from one person to another. Majority of athletes use powerlifting exercises to help increase their explosiveness and speed in addition to improving their vertical jump.

Powerlifting is important for athletes who want to compete on a high level. When you participate in ultra long distance swimming, biking, or running, you are doing repetitive movement that is more prone to over use injury. When you do strength training, you break up that movement and improve your ability to recover from injuries; you also improve your ability to prevent those injuries. When you constantly overuse certain muscle groups within your body, other muscle groups do not work. This leads to joint instability, as well as other problems. Powerlifting really helps athletes improve their core strength, hip strength, leg and back strength, as well as shoulder strength. Athletes will compete on a high level of intensity, which means that you will sacrifice your body, and you will not remain in the best health at times. However, it is important that you do not sacrifice your lean mass, which powerlifting helps you avoid.

It is worth noting that not all endurance athletes were born endurance athletes. The same is true with many other athletes, including powerlifters. These individuals had to devote a lot of time to themselves, preparing their body to handle the mental, physical, and emotional aspects of a sport. It is true that people that are new to a sport do not know how to properly train for that sport. However, with the proper coaching and a determination to succeed, they can learn all what they need to compete on a high level.

A person who was born to endure all will likely have the sport down to a science. High level athletes are very in tune with their bodies and know what is necessary to do in order to achieve success. However, someone who is new to sports may not know where to begin, and that is okay. Strength training will help you learn what is necessary to not only compete within the sport, but to compete successfully.

Sports that are more endurance-based do not require as much strength more than other sports. A high level of strength is not required for the sports that are endurance-based. However, there are some sports that require explosive power and speed. Sports that are more explosive in nature require a higher level of strength than endurance sports. Sports such as wrestling and football would fall under this category. Lastly, there are sports that require pure strength. Sports like weightlifting and powerlifting would fall into this category. Powerlifting is the sport that requires a lot of strength, but not a lot of other qualities. Those athletes that run track will need speed for the 40 and 50 meter dash, while someone who participates in the shot throw or baseball will need more power. Baseball players will also need speed as well as a host of other athletic qualities, but a track runner will require pure speed and power to compete.

Football players and wrestlers need more power to compete at a high level and in turn a higher level of strength. These types of athletes will need more strength and power, in comparison to someone who is a long distance runner. Lacrosse is more of an endurance type sport as compared to football, which requires shorter bursts of athletic activity. Wrestlers will need to lift people off of the ground, but runners need more speed and endurance. When using strength training as a means to get better in sport it is important to understand what qualities are necessary to compete at a high level so you can gauge how much strength you really need. That being said becoming stronger will never hurt the cause no matter what sport you engage in!

The training for an athlete is important, regardless of what sport they play. One of the biggest mistakes that many parents and coaches make is allowing the trainees to go straight into plyometrics and speed training before they have developed the muscle mass or any foundation of strength. Think about the way your car runs; if you do not have an engine, will it move very fast? No! This is why an athlete that gains more muscle mass and gets stronger will have the potential for more speed later down the road. Those athletes that do not have a great deal of muscle mass to begin with will not be able as explosive and fast, even when doing extensive speed training because they don't have a big enough foundation due to their lack of strength.

One particular example that I have is about a wrestler. When I began training him, he was a tenth grade student; now, he is a senior at Harvard University. When he began, he had a lot of potential, and I knew with the proper training, he could become great. He was a heavy kid, but after training, he had placed as the number three wrestler in the county. This was an extremely competitive weight class, and the fact that he placed was very impressive for a tenth grade student. The bigger an athlete is, the more strength he or she will need to have. By the time this student reached his junior year of high school, he was not only winning all of the counties in his division, but he placed at the state level as well. During his senior year, the athlete had placed within the states, and he had won the counties again, but in a higher and more competitive weight class.

Since this athlete, David, was competing at such a high level, he was able to start on the Division I level at his college. He is now the starting heavyweight for his wrestling team and has been for all four years of schooling. When I met him, I knew that he had potential, but he was not very strong at the time. He had not really dialed in the technique, but through strength training, he realized his true power, and his true potential. It is difficult to come onto a team as a freshman and start as a heavyweight, especially at a Division I school. David not only started as heavyweight during his freshman year, but he had this honor for the next three years as well. Another accomplishment that he had was being All Conference twice, and qualifting for the NCAA tournament.

David is one of the success stories that I love telling. It was not only his accomplishments that make his story so special, but it was his commitment and dedication that make me proud. He is a true example of what strength training can do for an individual, and an athlete. He not only trained during the in-season, but he trained during off-season too. He did not take time off; he was truly focused. Often I see countless athletes take time off and not engage in their training as much as they should. When they stop training, they lose their strength, which is never a good thing. Having strength counts, and when you do, you can accomplish those goals that you have set for yourself.

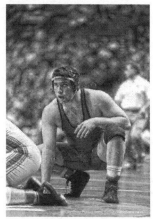

"I started training with John Gaglione in the summer, going into tenth grade. I was just recently brought up to varsity football, and after hearing a lot about the success of the guys he had trained; I figured that training with him would be a great idea. I originally trained with him to become a very good football player. During my sophomore wrestling season, I trained with Coach Gaglione, and I feel that it was his doing that really got me into wrestling. I continued to train consistently with him right through my senior wrestling season. Coach Gaglione played a huge part in helping me win two section 8 wrestling titles and going all state twice; he always pushed me to train and improve, even when I did not want to. He always pushed me to be the best that I could; training with him has really paid dividends. My strength, flexibility, and over all athleticism has improved greatly since I have been with him. I plan to continue training with John throughout my college wrestling career. Training with him has been great and I attribute much of my success to him." – *Two Time County Champion, Two Time All State NCAA Qualifier Harvard University Wrestler David Ng*

Another example is a female athlete that I helped train. I began training her when she was a senior in high school. Unlike the previous example, this young lady was very accomplished. She was an All Long Island softball player and pitcher, but she had a lot of issues pertaining to her shoulders and other similar areas. She did not realize her own power. When her college strength coach sent her packets for strength and conditioning, she was confused and didn't know where to start. She had no idea what she was supposed to do. This is when she enlisted my help in order to get stronger. During her strength training, we did a lot of different powerlifting movements, in addition to weightlifting movements. Due to her strength training and commitment, she went on to pitch all four years during her Division I collegiate career. She began throwing harder and even helped lead her team to a couple of championship titles. She was named to the All Conference team multiples times while in college, while leading her team win back to back conference championships.

When she came to me, I knew that she needed to get stronger. She needed to improve her squat strength, as well as her deadlift strength. Doing so allowed her to improve her hip power, which allowed her to be more explosive and throw harder. She was strong enough to be a starting Division I pitcher, which is exactly what she did. Even though she came to me as an accomplished athlete, the training she received helped take her to that next level. She was able to realize her true potential, and she reached her goal of being a competitive collegiate athlete.

These are just two of the many examples that I have pertaining to powerlifting, and how it works for athletes in general. When these two athletes came to me, they improved their strength, and they decreased the amount of injuries they had over the years. Their athletics qualities improved as a result of the strength training. Powerlifting movements aren't just reserved for high-level athletes; it is training that benefits all athletes who want to become stronger and excel in their sport.

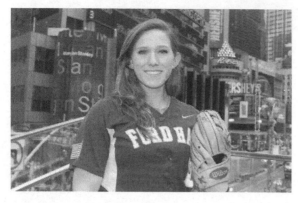 "I began working with Coach Gaglione in the summer after my senior year of high school after having heard of the work Coach Gaglione had done with many of the top male athletes at Plainedge High School, and the significant gains they had made on the playing field as a result of his training. Seeing as my first season of division I softball began only three months later, I was eager to start training with Coach Gaglione because I knew he had the knowledge and the skills to help me succeed at the next level. Now having trained with him for an extended period of time, I can say that I am beyond grateful for all that he has done, as I have made significant physical gains ranging from improved strength and flexibility to increased explosiveness, all of which have transcended to my

ability on the field. I attribute all of my success both in the

gym and on the field to Coach Gaglione. He constantly

motivates all of his athletes, myself included, to go beyond

their limits to attain each and every goal they set out to

fulfill." – *All Long Island All Conference at Fordam*

University Softball Player Michele Daubman

Chapter 5: Using Powerlifting to Build Muscle

Over the years, I have worked with many individuals that want to build muscle. It is true that powerlifting can help build muscle with athletes, as well as non-athletes. When you focus more on strength training, the result is stronger, bigger, and more defined muscles. This means dropping any unnecessary workouts that do not work, and replace them with the training that does. More isn't always better. Better is better. The key is to find the optimal amount of work, and number of exercises that works for you to achieve your personal goals. When you focus on the three lifts (squats, bench press, and deadlifts), you will work out your entire body. The end result is building thick muscles, without the need of special exercise equipment or <>machines.

Powerlifting gives you a strong foundation because it literally works out every single muscle that is in your body. These heavy compound movements are what give you overall strength, as well as a well-rounded physique. Many people make the mistake of doing isolation movements too soon. When they want bigger arms, they stick to doing curls all of the time. The problem with this is that they do not have any base strength; it is not possible to use an optimal weight due to the fact that they are not strong enough. When you are stronger, you are able to use a higher amount of weight, and you can do a higher number of sets with a higher weight. This will improve your volume, in addition to your time under tension. This ultimately leads to increased muscle growth, which increases your size and your lean body mass. With added strength training, you will become bigger, more athletic, and your physique will be more balanced.

I am not saying that isolation is something you can never do; I am stating that you need to get stronger before you can use heavy weights with your isolation. For beginners, I suggest starting out and focusing on learning the basic compound movements. Your main focus should be to work on your strength and learning technique in the classic lifts and basic exercises. Learning to squat, push, pull, and hip hinge are critical skills for everyone to learn, regardless of what their goals are. At the beginning of your workout, you will need more motor units and more of your nervous system, which is why the heavy compound movements and powerlifts should be performed first. After you finish your compound movements, there is nothing wrong with moving on to isolation movements. Once you reach a certain level, isolation movements can be very helpful in brining up weak points and attacking the specific body parts that you want to grow.

Powerlifting does a great job of giving you good awareness of your body. It is very important to have body awareness when you want to focus on contracting certain muscles. When you have good mind-muscle connection, powerlifting can teach you how to:

- Use your full body as a unit
- Use your core strength
- Engage certain muscle groups for stability
- Be more in tune with your body in order to activate your muscular fibers

Powerlifting does a great job of helping you target the muscles in your body that you want to work. A common mistake is using a lot of momentum, when you need to be using your muscle to move the weight. This is a huge problem that powerlifting can help with. Powerlifting is slower and more controlled, allowing you to truly engage your muscles. It is extremely important that you engage your muscle instead of using momentum. When you use momentum to move weight instead of muscle, you are never going to grow. This is why powerlifting is really important when it pertains to building size and increasing your lean mass.

Testimonial:

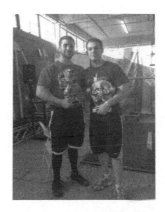

"After never touching a weight for the first 21 years of my life, powerlifting became the driving force behind both my career and personal growth. Powerlifting has provided the basis of which I derive my training techniques as a strength coach, and a personal trainer. In my personal life, it's been the catalyst for improving my health, physique, and self-confidence. It's hard to imagine that any other sport could have such a positive impact on so many facets of my life. I know that anyone could reap the same benefits from powerlifting that I have been fortunate enough to experience." *- Robert Riccobono*

Chapter 6: Powerlifting and the Elderly

We have already discussed how powerlifting is something that people can do, regardless of shape and size. This also applies to most ages. Powerlifting is something that elderly individuals can do; in fact, powerlifting has many benefits for everyone, including senior citizens. Powerlifting is highly recommended for elderly individuals.

It is true that men over the age of 60 are able to increase their strength by 80 percent due to powerlifting. Some researchers report that older men gain strength at the same rate as men in their 20s. An Ohio study showed that men between the ages of 60-75 who had no previous strength training were 50 to 80 percent stronger after completing a 16 week powerlifting training program. This particular study also showed improvement in the seniors' aerobic capacity, cholesterol profile, and muscle tone.

Powerlifting has been able to help both male and female seniors. Some studies show that changes in the strength and muscle size in senior citizens were similar to those conducted on college-age individuals. This backs up the theory that no age can truly limit a person's ability to get stronger from strength training. This is why powerlifting is beneficial, and recommended, for seniors. I want to stress the importance of building muscle mass as we age. As you get older, your body will start to lose it's muscle mass overtime. This can have negative impact on your health. It is important for us all to maintain a certain amount of muscle mass as we grow older in age.

Powerlifting also has a positive impact on the cardiovascular system of elderly individuals. After powerlifting, tests have shown that seniors use oxygen more efficiently. After strength training, it takes seniors longer to reach that point of exhaustion, which is a good thing.

Powerlifting has been known to improve the cholesterol levels of seniors who participate in powerlifting. When blood samples have been taken from seniors who lifted, their LDL cholesterol levels have been reported to decrease, while their HDL cholesterol levels increase. It is true that if elderly individuals maintain a certain level of strength training through exercise and powerlifting, their quality of life will be better as they age.

It is always a good idea to hire a coach when powerlifting, especially if you are older in age. A coach can help you learn the proper weight lifting techniques and strength training workouts. It is also a good idea to consult with a physician before beginning any type of weight lifting regimen.

Testimonial:

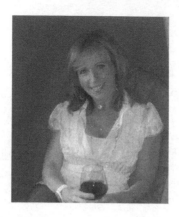

I have been active my whole life, gymnastics, aerobics, yoga...And my job . All took a toll on my back. I've been suffering for years with back pain. My daughter Danielle joined 2 years ago, and I watched her body transform, she looks amazing. I'm 54 and never thought about lifting, though it would hurt me even more. Well was I wrong!!! She convinced me to join; now, four months later, I can't even tell you how great I feel.

My back is almost 100% better. John told me that you have to keep moving, especially when you get older, and he was right...I look forward to every class and cant wait to see how I look in the months to come....

John has been such a great coach and I thank him for helping me." – *Carole Kay*

Chapter 7: Powerlifting Beyond Sports

Powerlifting has helped people who participate in sports, but this type of strength training is also great for the non-athlete. There are many people who participate in powerlifting to help improve their overall mental state. There is a competitive edge and mental strength that comes with powerlifting. I discussed briefly how strength goes beyond your power and lifting abilities; it is also determined by your mental and emotional state. Having a stronger body can in turn help give you a stronger mind and spirit as well.

Strength training is extremely beneficial to your mental health. Studies have shown that strength training helps with a variety of mental health issues, including:

- Anxiety

- Fatigue

- Self-Esteem

- Depression

- Sleep

- Chronic Pain

- Cognition

- and more…

Strength training helps your mental health because it causes morphological adaptations, as well as neural adaptations. Strength training has a positive effect on the mental health through changes that take place in your brain. Strength training has the ability to help us overcome mental challenges, just as much as we can overcome physical challenges. Powerlifting gives you the will and mental resolve to overcome those challenges.

If you have ever been a part of a group at school, or a team at work, you know that there is a certain amount of stress that goes with those groups and teams. Strength training can help with those emotional issues. In fact, powerlifting has been known to help people with their emotional state pertaining to daily routines. You can help build your self-esteem and confidence through strength training. When people are unhappy with their appearance, this has a negative effect on them emotionally.

Powerlifting strength is measured by the amount of weight on the bar. While physique changes may take time to happen strength changes can happen in a matter of weeks especially if you are a beginner. When trainees see their improvement and see the weight on the bar increase, it takes away the stress of them always focusing on physical appearance, and it can boost their confidence and self esteem through improved performance. Through powerlifting, you can improve your physique as well as your performance, which could give you a huge emotional lift.

The endorphins released during strength training also help improve your emotional state. The chemicals released from your brain can stimulate feelings of happiness. When you are happy and stress free, these chemicals are typically released. Powerlifting has a positive way of helping you relieve the stress that you may feel at home, school, or work. Once you have completed a weight lifting session at the gym or your home, you will feel happy and accomplished. This positivity is due to the endorphins that have been released.

Testimonial:

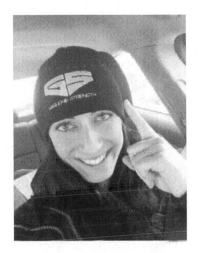

"Sports have always been a microcosm of my life. But even though a "small world" within my world, it IS my world. My lifting comes out in the strength needed through my life, and my life comes out in my lifting. Harboring any internal battles through the focus of my lift. The very definition of myself comes through the resilience I have created and reinforced by my sport.

I met John Gaglione and was introduced to Gaglione Strength while attending a workshop in his facility. I didn't know walking in that day how much my future as a trainer would improve, or how much I'd grow and change as an individual.

Quick to welcome me on board, John patiently worked with me as I got started. Although everyone is serious about their work and lifts at Gaglione, there is a sense of family, community, and everyone is willing to help and share their knowledge. In the fitness industry, as a whole, there is always someone hoping you don't do as well as them, or hoping that you fall on your face. But in this close knit atmosphere, the support is abundant and genuine. I wouldn't have accomplished some of the things I have without the G team.

When I think about strength training and power lifting, I think of all strong willed people, and those who aren't satisfied with the mediocrity that our lives can hold until you push the envelope a little. You can't be satisfied with "settling" in life, or in lifting. If you settle, you have failed. If you accept that you've made it as far as you can go, or believe that you won't get stronger, or you won't accomplish your goal, you have failed. The potential we have is far greater than we give ourselves credit for. In powerlifting, there's always something more to discover about yourself and improve upon. The perseverance to your goal and potential requires patience.

Mental toughness is one of the only things that matters to me, pertaining to improving myself and my clients. I've had friends pass away, and seen relationships die, but I have to stay as positive as my mind will allow. I choose what I allow in, but someone will always have it worse than you, and they need the mental toughness even more to fight through it. If you can check the anger, sadness, or cruelty of the world at the door, and fuel your fire with those emotions, you'll burn through the workout and lifts. If you push through these times, you can truly conquer your life. There is no second chance in your life, and there's no second chance to perform at your absolute best. Every day, give it everything that you got. Lifting teaches you that some days it won't all come together, but when it does, the harmony of your body and the barbell is enough to change your whole world around. This may sound like a stretch to some, but I challenge everyone to find something that does this for you. If you haven't moved any heavy weight, then maybe it is time to try it.

Life is hard, and being happy by society's definition is harder. We must define our own lives, and our own terms of what it means to be happy. We have to give and take all of the time, and I know that I was given a gift leaving Gaglione's, after one of the first few sessions. I had been so caught up in my bodybuilding workouts that I was losing myself in the process. I wasn't enjoying my workouts. I used to wait with excitement all day to lift, and I was beginning to see that fade. Powerlifting gave me a new purpose, and put the fun and "point" back into why I was working out. It's not just about what my body looks like. It should never be just about that. That feeling will fade like an untrue love. It's how unstoppable I feel knowing that I can conquer what's before me, and move this weight that's about to bear down on me.

I was losing that same mental toughness and focus that carried me through some of the hardest times of my life. I often sat wondering with fear and frustration about what I could possibly do to improve myself again. After my second time deadlifting at Gaglione's, my life found what it was missing. And on the long drive back to my house, I knew I was all in, and coming out of the dark shadow I'd been in." - *Gianna Masi*

Chapter 8: Should you Compete

When you hear the word powerlifting, you may automatically think about competing. It is true that some people sign up for strength training to receive help with weight loss, as well as mental and emotional health improvement. I believe that all powerlifters should, at the very least, try to compete, but that is a decision that you need to make on your own. Many people are surprised to see how fun and rewarding competing can be once they give it a try.

After you have decided that competing is something you want to do, you should know when it is the right time to compete. A coach can help you determine if you are ready to compete, and at what level you are ready to compete at.

The rules associated with powerlifting will vary because there are different powerlifting federations. This is why a great coach will help you prepare for those rules, as well as the different atmospheres and lifters. Some powerlifting competitions allow you to use equipment, while some do not. This is one reason why you want to practice strength training without machines. Equipment may include:

- Weight Lifting Belts

- Squat Suits

- Knee Wraps/Sleeves

- Bench Press Shirts

- Wrist Wraps

- and more…

If you prefer to enter competitions that allow the use of equipment, you should know what type of equipment is acceptable prior to your meet. Most lifting gear is approved for meets, but you should still verify that this is true.

All powerlifting atmospheres are different. Regardless of how many years you have been competing, this fact will never change. Some meets will have loud music playing in the background, while other meets will have no music at all. Cheering for teams and teammates takes place during some meets, which can be a huge distraction if you are not mentally prepared.

When the time comes for you to compete, a judge will yell out to you. The meet promoter may yell something like, "You are on deck!" At this time, you will need to unleash your very best. All of the adrenaline in your body will kick in, and the eyes of the crowd will be placed onto you. The atmosphere is generally very intense at this time. It is extremely important that you contain your composure. This level of intensity could have you doing things that you did not do during normal training, such as pushing yourself to higher weights. Do not allow the fire burning inside of your chest to push you past your current limits; do what you have practiced doing. Of course, sometimes advanced lifters who are trying to win a national level competition will need to take calculated risks and push the envelop a little bit more, but even in these advanced cases, 90% of the time it is best to stick to your planned attempt, and only adjust marginally, based on how you are feeling that day, and based on how the previous attempts looked and felt on the platform. Use the extra intensity to stay focused and stick to your game plan. This is why it is important to have a coach. It can be very easy to let your emotions get the best of you. A coach will allow you to just focus on the execution of the lift so you don't need to worry as much about strategy or weight attempts. Emotions can cloud your judgments, especially when the competition is fierce.

I always tell my trainees to get a good night's rest before competing. The week up until the competition you want to take it easy. Some athletes decide not to train at all, which is acceptable. On the day of your competition, a good rule of thumb is to eat a breakfast that is high in carbohydrates with moderate protein and low in fat. This gives you energy. If you want to boost your energy levels, you can drink some caffeine before each event. Most people have small meals throughout the day, before and after each of the events, while staying hydrated throughout the day. These are just some general guidelines and of course it is important to NOT try anything drastically different than what you normally do in training. Eat how you normally eat, and only take in what your body is used to. If you try something different, you won't know how your body is going to react.

Remember to always remain positive on the day of your competition. During the day, think of positive thoughts. Let the confidence that you have during your training sessions carry out onto the powerlifting platform.

All good things must come to an end, and powerlifting competitions are one of those things. You must know when it is time to compete, and you must also know when it is time to retire. The fact is, it is never too late to begin powerlifting. Athletes that are older 40s can still compete at a high level, just like a teenager. You probably have a lot more competitive years in you then you realize. You are competing to gain experience and to get better; therefore, everyone is just like you, which is why they are supportive during the competition. Remember that there are plenty of strong men and women that do not have the confidence to compete, so you are already accomplishing a big feat just by competing.

The answer to when it is time to retire will rely solely on you, and your body. Some people in their 70s and 80s have been known to deadlift some serious poundages; some even in the 400 lb range, which is why they may still compete. Normally, the ability to squat goes first, and then bench, followed by the deadlift last. This is due to the joints involved, and the range of motion required for each lift. This is a passion that could turn into a lifelong hobby, but when your body is no longer able to lift at a consistent level or you are in too much pain to lift with good form, you will need to retire from competitions.

Before it is time to retire, know your limits and how often you should compete. A beginner competitor shouldn't worry about competing too often and just worry about getting a few contests in per year to get their feet wet. Intermediate lifters can compete three times, and highly advanced lifters can complete once at a national level or world competitive and usually one other time to qualify for their big contest. During the off season, a powerlifter should train and work on weak links and look to improve their work capacity and increase their training volumes.

Testimonial:

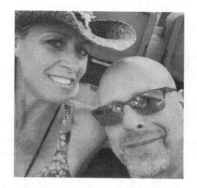

"I am so glad I took that first step and began strength training with my teenage son's peers and girls who were more than 20 years younger than me. I am comfortable in the gym and no longer fear the "big barbell". I would say, thanks to John's guidance I have a pretty decent squat, bench, and deadlift. I feel and look stronger than ever.

I hope to call myself a competitive powerlifter by the time I turn 50; something I never expected to put on my bucket list! I am enjoying my training every step of the way." *– Andrea Loconte*

Chapter 9: What Type of Diet Should a Powerlifter Have?

While it is true that some big time powerlifters in the past do not follow a proper diet, this is something that you should avoid doing. More and more high-level powerlifters are turning toward better nutrition programs to aid in their performance. Proper nutrition is not only good for athletes, but it is necessary to have good health overall. Do not eat more portions just to gain weight; this is an unhealthy habit. The healthier you eat while strength training, the better you will feel. Failing to follow a good diet could cause you to feel sluggish. People who follow a proper diet are known to have more energy when powerlifting.

One thing I will say, just like with training, everyone is different and our bodies respond differently to different diets and foods, which is why it is important to work with a coach if you really want to take your performance to the next level. That being said, here are some basic guidelines to follow in order to help you get started.

Fats may be considered bad for the average person, but when you understand how fats truly work in your body, you will realize that fats are an important part of your diet. You should never go too low fat; not allowing yourself to go below a 20 percent fat intake on your diet is a good rule of thumb. You should avoid saturated fats, and trans fats.

Carbohydrates have also gained a bad reputation over the years, but the truth is, you need them. Just like fats, there are good and bad carbs. The carbs that are full of fiber are good for your heart, and they help control your blood sugar levels. In order to lose body fat, you will need to keep your blood sugar levels under control. A good rule of thumb is to have more carbs around your training time and during workout days. More intense workouts require more fuel. If you aren't training on a particular day you don't need as many carbs.

Protein is very important when it pertains to supporting muscle tissue. If one of your goals is to gain muscle, you will need to consume plenty of protein within your diet. The best forms of protein to eat are lean proteins. It is a misconception that shakes are the only source of protein that you should have. It is important that you receive protein from food sources as well. Shakes are great when you are on the go or if you have a hard time eating solid food right after a workout. As an athlete hitting your protein and fiber targets should always be a top priority. A good rule of thumb is to have a lean source of protein with each meal to ensure you are getting enough protein each day. Ultra high protein diets aren't necessary, but I have found most of the general population under-eat protein, and usually overeat on carbs, fat, or both. It is rarer to see someone overeat on lean protein, which is why many coaches put an emphasis on it.

When you develop a good diet; stick to it. An example of the proper diet would be:

- 4- 6 meals per day as it fits your lifestyle

- Look to have low glycemic carbs earlier in the day

- Higher glycemic carbs closer to workout time (pre, post)

- Aim for around 1 gram of bodyweight protein, per pound of lean body weight

- Higher Fat on non training days

- Higher Carb on Training days

Testimonial:

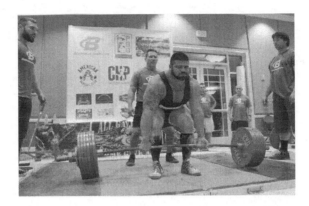

"Powerlifting has become a huge part of my life. I can honestly say I might be obsessed with it. I started off as a guy who really didn't train hard, nor take it too serious, but I managed to get the same results in return. Things changed for me when I went to watch Raw Unity 7. I have seen the best in the world, in-person, and I realized that although these guys and girls were super strong, they were regular people just like me. So when I got home, things changed: nutrition, training, and my mindset. I went from an 1840 total, to 2000 raw in 5 short months. I also found out through being a member at Gaglione strength what a team meant, and that I loved helping and coaching as well.

My passion of powerlifting is growing more and more each day, and I won't stop 'till I physically can't do it anymore." - *Dom Minnici*

Conclusion

One of the best things about powerlifting is the fact that it is black and white. If your total goes up, the program has been a success, and you have gotten stronger. It is that simple. You have put in a specific amount of dedication, hard work, and made sacrifices in order to achieve your goals. The feeling that you receive from this accomplishment is indescribable, but it is great for your mental and emotional state, as well as your physical state.

It is not necessary for you to compete on an athletic level when you sign up for powerlifting, but I suggest that you try. If you are like me, once you have that iron bug, you will not want to stop. When I began powerlifting at the age of 17, I never imagined that I would open my own gym and train a team of nationally ranked powerlifters, but I have.

If you are on the fence about starting strength training and powerlifting, I hope after reading this book you sincerely give this a try. Powerlifting is a gift that has made a huge impact on my life, and it has made me the man that I am today. The inner strength you gain, and the relationships you will build while embarking on yours strength training journey will allow you to soar to new heights that you never thought were possible. It has allowed me an outlet to help empower so many people so that in turn, they can reach their personal goals. My mission is to help build a stronger community, one more person at a time, so even if this book only inspires one person to get started, I will consider that a success.

Regardless of why you choose to sign up for strength training, you should always seek out a good coach. A great coach will help you train properly, ensuring that you are on the right track to achieve your goals! I invite you to seriously give an honest effort to starting a strength training program. It might sound cliché, but this can truly be life changing.

About the Author

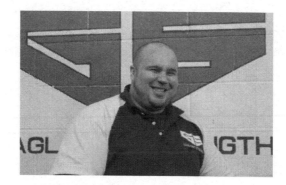

John Gaglione is a strength coach based out of Long Island, New York. John trains people from all walks of life at his facility, which is located in Farmingdale, New York. He specializes in improving maximal strength for athletes and "average Joes". John coaches a powerlifting team that consists of more than 40 lifters; over 20 of those lifters hold national ranking in their respective weight classes and divisions.

John has written many strength and conditioning articles for major online publications, such as *Men's Health, Elite Fitness Systems, Testosterone Nation, One Result,* and he is the featured strength & conditioning author for *Long Island Wrestling Association.* John has been a featured speaker at several schools, including Cortland and Hofstra Universities – for their exercise science programs.

As an avid strength athlete, John also has a lot of "under the bar experience," and he has competed in the sport of powerlifting for over a decade. He has the best competition lifts: an 850 Squat, 575 Bench, and a 640 Deadlift.

If you would like to learn more about John, you can reach him at gaglionestrength@gmail.com.

Train With Gaglione Strength

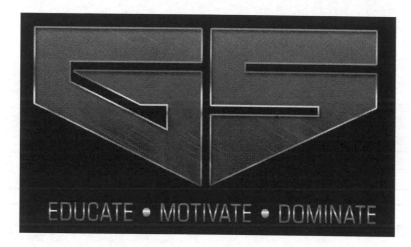

For locals you can request a complimentary session by sending an e-mail to gaglionestrength@gmail.com with the subject line "powerlifting for the people" and we will get your scheduled for your session.

For those who are not in the Tri-state area, you can take full advantage of our Elite Distance Coaching program by going to: http://www.gaglionestrength.com/online-training/

<No matter where you are or what level you are at we can help you get to the next one and help you become the strongest version of you! >

Made in the USA
Lexington, KY
27 October 2015